How To Get Rid Of Eczema Quickly

294 Great Tips For Eczema Relief

ADAM COLTON

Published by BizMove
www.bizmove.com

Table of Contents

1. Eczema Fact Sheet

A combination of genetic and environmental factors appears to be involved in the development of eczema. The condition often is associated with other allergic diseases such as asthma, hay fever, and food allergy. Children whose parents have asthma and allergies are more likely to develop atopic dermatitis than children of parents without allergic diseases. Approximately 30 percent of children with atopic dermatitis have food allergies, and many develop asthma or respiratory allergies. People who live in cities or drier climates also appear more likely to develop the disease.

The condition tends to worsen when a person is exposed to certain triggers, such as

- Pollen, mold, dust mites, animals, and certain foods (for allergic individuals)
- Cold and dry air
- Colds or the flu
- Skin contact with irritating chemicals
- Skin contact with rough materials such as wool
- Emotional factors such as stress

- Fragrances or dyes added to skin lotions or soaps.

Taking too many baths or showers and not moisturizing the skin properly afterward may also make eczema worse.

Skin Care at Home

You and your doctor should discuss the best treatment plan and medications for your atopic dermatitis. But taking care of your skin at home may reduce the need for prescription medications. Some recommendations include

- Avoid scratching the rash or skin.
- Relieve the itch by using a moisturizer or topical steroids. Take antihistamines to reduce severe itching.
- Keep your fingernails cut short. Consider light gloves if nighttime scratching is a problem.
- Lubricate or moisturize the skin two to three times a day using ointments such as petroleum jelly. Moisturizers should be free of alcohol, scents, dyes, fragrances, and other skin-irritating chemicals. A humidifier in the home also can help.
- Avoid anything that worsens symptoms, including

- o Irritants such as wool and lanolin (an oily substance derived from sheep wool used in some moisturizers and cosmetics)
  - o Strong soaps or detergents
  - o Sudden changes in body temperature and stress, which may cause sweating
- When washing or bathing
  - o Keep water contact as brief as possible and use gentle body washes and cleansers instead of regular soaps. Lukewarm baths are better than long, hot baths.
  - o Do not scrub or dry the skin too hard or for too long.
  - o After bathing, apply lubricating ointments to damp skin. This will help trap moisture in the skin.

Wet Wrap Therapy

Researchers at NIAID and other institutions are studying an innovative treatment for severe eczema called wet wrap therapy. It includes three lukewarm baths a day, each followed by an application of topical medicines and moisturizer that is sealed in by a wrap of wet gauze.

People with severe eczema have come to the National Institutes of Health Clinical Center in Bethesda, Maryland, for research evaluation.

Treatment may include wet wrap therapy to bring the condition under control. Patients and their caregivers also receive training on home-based skin care to properly manage flare-ups once they leave the hospital.

Eczema (Atopic Dermatitis) Complications

The skin of people with atopic dermatitis lacks infection-fighting proteins, making them susceptible to skin infections caused by bacteria and viruses. Fungal infections also are common in people with atopic dermatitis.

Bacterial Infections

A major health risk associated with atopic dermatitis is skin colonization or infection by bacteria such as *Staphylococcus aureus*. Sixty to 90 percent of people with atopic dermatitis are likely to have staph bacteria on their skin. Many eventually develop infection, which worsens the atopic dermatitis.

Viral Infections

People with atopic dermatitis are highly vulnerable to certain viral infections of the skin. For example, if infected with herpes simplex virus, they can develop a severe skin condition called atopic dermatitis with eczema herpeticum.

Those with atopic dermatitis should not receive the currently licensed smallpox vaccine, even if their disease is in remission, because they are at risk of developing a severe infection called eczema vaccinatum. This infection is caused when the live vaccinia virus in the smallpox vaccine reproduces and spreads throughout the body. Furthermore, those in close contact with people who have atopic dermatitis or a history of the disease should not receive the smallpox vaccine because of the risk of transmitting the live vaccine virus to the person with atopic dermatitis.

2. 294 Great Tips For Eczema Relief

If you want to learn more about coping with eczema then this book is going to discuss some important topics for your benefit. As you continue to read, focus on the facts about this type of skin condition and what you can do. As with everything, the more you know the better off you are.

1. Dress in cotton, or at least wear a cotton blend. This type of fabric usually does not irritate people who have eczema. Avoid things like polyester, which can cause an outbreak. In addition, when you purchase new clothing, make sure you put it in the washing machine prior to wearing it.

2. When buying a detergent, look for something that is not scented. If you are having trouble finding one that works for you, look for products labeled "free and clear" and see if they work. In addition, it may be best not to use a fabric softener at all. This product can cause an issue for people with eczema, so it is usually not worth the risk.

3. Be careful when you put on sunscreen. You never know what may cause you to have an outbreak of eczema. The higher the SPF, the more likely it is that the sunscreen may cause you to have an issue. Try and find something with an SPF of around 35. That should protect your skin from the sun and keep it in good shape overall.

4. If you suffer with eczema flare-ups, be sure that your skin remains moisturized. That will help you manage your symptoms better. Particularly when you get out of the shower, put on a little moisturizer. Do not use moisturizers that contain fragrances or scents.

5. When selecting a moisturizer look for ointments. They are better at soothing eczema because of their ability to seal in moisture by providing a protective layer. Lotions and other creams you might be using aren't going to provide this soothing relief. Therefore, ointments are better for eczema.

6. Help prevent eczema flare ups by keeping skin moisturized. When skin is moisturized, it is soft and pliable, thus reducing cracking. Petroleum jelly or unscented moisturizers with a few simple ingredients are best. Some moisturizers have chemicals and fragrances and will aggravate eczema instead of relieving it.

7. Get in the bath if you feel an eczema break-out coming on. Not only does the bath add some much needed moisture to your skin, but it also is needed to remove debris and irritants that may be causing the break out. Don't add oils or perfumes to the bath.

8. When taking a bath or shower, use only very gentle cleansers. Don't scrub too hard. After you take a shower or a bath, pat your skin dry gently. Be sure to moisturize all over with a natural oil such as olive oil. This will help keep the moisture from your bath in your skin.

9. How you bathe is important if you suffer from eczema. For starters, stay away from hot showers or baths; this will just irritate your skin. Use water that is room temperature. Do not scrub your skin and stay away from scented soaps. When you are done showering, pat your skin dry.

10. Instead of scratching, try using ice to cool itchy areas. You can get an inexpensive gel compress and keep it in the freezer. Take it out and hold it over itchy areas whenever you need to. Keep a dry washcloth in your purse or pocket at all times. If you become very itchy away from home, soak the cloth in cold water. Hold it over the itchy area.

11.   Avoid scrubbing your skin. Eczema won't just scrub away in the shower. Scrubbing your skin when you bathe will only serve to irritate it. Avoid using exfoliating scrubs and rough sponges or loofahs. Instead, use cotton rags and a gentle, unscented soap for sensitive skin. This will be much easier on your skin.

12.   Consider getting rid of your carpets and throw rugs throughout your house. Carpet and rugs are known for harboring dust mites, allergens and other microscopic irritants which can cause an eczema flair-up. So consider hardwood floors or a low pile carpet if you absolutely must have carpet in your house.

13.   Use a wet cloth to dust. This grabs the dust, and it sticks to the rag. Dry dusting causes the dust to affect the air you breath.

14.   When taking a bath, don't use excessively hot water. It will dry out your skin which will aggravate your eczema. Use warm water, a gentle soap and a soft rag to clean any patches of eczema that you have. If you really want to use a loofah or a scrubbie then only use it on unaffected areas and rinse, clean and dry the loofah or scrubbie afterwards.

15.   Always apply a moisturizer or lotion after taking a bath or shower. Your skin will have absorbed moisture and using a moisturizer or lotion after a bath or shower will help to keep that moisture locked in your skin. So keep a long lasting lotion on hand and use it as part of your bath ritual.

16.   Find a sunscreen that works for you. Getting a sunburn is terrible for your skin. At the same time, certain sunscreens can make eczema worse. It is important that you experiment with different sunscreens before using one. Find a sunscreen that will protect your skin from the sun without irritating it.

17.   Watch out for very tight clothing. Tighter clothes can irritate the skin needlessly. You are more likely to experience an eczema episode. You want to wear clothing that is loose and comfortable. This will reduce the sweat that your body produces.

18.   Taking certain supplements is great for those suffering from eczema. Most people simply do not get the nutrients they need from the foods they eat everyday; this is why taking supplements is beneficial. Fatty acids can decrease inflammation and relieve dry skin, while vitamins A,D,and E hydrate the skin and give it a better texture.

19.   Common treatments for eczema include topical creams and ointments that contain cortisone. You could try hydrocortisone that can be purchased at your local drug store. If this doesn't soothe your eczema, you should talk with your doctor about possibly getting a stronger prescription from him. These will work like other steroid creams, but will be able to be used for a longer time.

20.   If you have been prescribed medicine for your eczema, take it as directed. When all else fails, your doctor may be able to help ease your symptoms by prescribing you something a little stronger than what you can get over the counter. While no one really wants to rely on medication, sometimes it is necessary.

21.   Moisturize regularly. Moisturizers can help quite a bit when you're dealing with something like eczema. Use a moisturizer after your shower. Your moisturizer should not contain fragrances, chemicals, or other additives. These things can irritate the skin. Creams and lotions with a thick texture work best.

22.   Resist the urge to scratch. Scratching will only intensify that itchy feeling. It can also cause harm to your skin, including infection. Find other ways to

relieve that itch. Use moisturizers, medications, cold compresses, and long soaks in the tub instead. These methods relieve your itch and make you feel better.

23.   Winter weather can cause eczema to worsen. Anytime your skin is exposed to frigid air, it needs a protective barrier to protect it from moisture loss. On any skin areas, such as the face or neck, be sure to heavily apply a moisturizer. Moisturizers will help you avoid dry and cracking skin because it locks in your skin's natural oils.

24.   Keep sweating to a minimum when experiencing a flare-up. Your eczema symptoms will not like sweat when it hits. If you are active, it is important to get cooled off as soon as you are finished with your physical activities. If possible, shower immediately after exercising.

25.   Dust can cause issues. Rather than dry dusting, use a damp dust method instead. This will help capture the dust, rather than simply spreading it around the home. Also, because rugs and carpets are a beacon for dust, try not to have them in the house if at all possible.

26.   Try to avoid taking hot baths and showers. The extreme temperatures of the water can actually

cause eczema flare-ups. The humidity and steam can also dry your skin out, which can make eczema uncomfortable. Try using water that is room temperature any time you shower or take a bath.

27.   Make sure the air is not too dry in your home, especially in the rooms you spend most of your time in. Dry air can cause break outs of eczema. If it is the heating season or you have particularly dry air in your home, you can fix that by putting a humidifier in those rooms.

28.   Because eczema can be caused or aggravated by certain materials, choose your clothing with care. Clothes made of wool or synthetic materials may inflame your skin. Choose clothing made of natural fibers, such as cotton. This is less likely to irritate your skin, and natural fibers allow your skin to breathe, making it less likely that you become overheated. Since heat and sweating can also aggravate eczema, choosing the right fabrics for your clothes is doubly important.

29.   Help manage eczema by installing a humidifier. Dry air especially during the winter can cause dry skin which in turn causes eczema. A humidifier will put moisture in the air so your skin won't get as dry.

30.   Eczema is characterized by dry, irritated skin. You can soothe dry skin by bathing with an unscented and mild soap. A pharmacist can direct you to the mildest varieties found at drugstores. After bathing in warm, not hot water, be sure to apply your moisturizer while your skin is damp which will help your skin retain moisture. If you make this your regular bathing routine you should see marked improvement in your eczema symptoms over time.

31.   Moisturize your skin immediately after taking a bath. Applying lotion to your skin soon after your bath helps to lock in the moisture and prevents your skin from drying too much. For the best results, use a intensive moisturizer that does not have added perfumes or dyes, which can dry your skin more.

32.   It is important to avoid too much stress if you suffer from eczema. Of course, having the skin condition can cause stress, as can life itself. But, a lot of stress increases flare-ups. If you find yourself getting stressed out, learn how to relax yourself. Yoga and meditation are two great ideas.

33.   If you dust your house, use a clean damp cloth. This will help the dust stick to the cloth. If the cloth

is not damp, you will only be moving the dust around, which can cause issues for your eczema.

34.   Avoid soaps. Soap is a very alkaline substance that is not suitable for sensitive skin. If you do not feel like water gets you clean enough, try a cleanser with a neutral pH balance. Soaps with added fragrance are even worse for your skin when you suffer from eczema.

35.   If you have allergies, being exposed to what you are allergic to may make your eczema worse. Eczema is not an allergy, but some common allergens that could trigger eczema are dairy products, eggs, wheat and tomatoes. Other things that could make your eczema flare up are pet dander, pollen, dust and mold.

36.   The cold weather can damage your skin, particularly the skin on your hands. When you are outside in the winter, make sure you put on a pair of gloves. In particular, either cotton gloves or leather gloves will work the best. Stay away from wool gloves, as they may hurt more than they will help you.

37.   Lotions and creams do not usually work as well as ointments. Ointments have a bit more oil in them, which generally helps them moisturize more

effectively. They are a little harder to apply than creams, however, but they are much better at adding a protective layer to the skin and easing your symptoms.

38.   Those who have eczema should not use a washcloth or body sponge when they are taking a bath or a shower. If you wash your body with such rough-surfaced items, the friction will irritate your skin. Skin irritation can lead to a flare-up of your eczema. To clean your body, simply use your hands to lather up.

39.   Make sure the clothing you wear won't irritate your skin. Some materials, particularly synthetics, can trigger outbreaks. Cotton is the best choice in fabrics to wear. You should also wash any new clothing before wearing it. To accomplish this, use a mild liquid detergent that is unscented, and do not use fabric softener.

40.   Keep your hands protected. Wear rubber gloves while washing dishes or performing another activity in which your hands are submersed in water. For further protection, wear cotton gloves underneath the rubber ones to reduce sweat and irritation. Use the cotton gloves while performing other activities, such as gardening and housework.

41.   Do not scratch your eczema. It is hard to resist because eczema is an itchy skin condition, but scratching makes it worse. You can increase the itching, damage your skin, and increase your risk of getting an infection. Try keeping the skin moisturized, bathing regularly, and using cold compresses to alleviate itching.

42.   Experiment with suntan lotions to find one that works for you. Certain sunscreens may exacerbate your eczema while others will not. However, what works for one person doesn't necessarily work for another. Keep trying them until you find one you can live with. However, be sure to just test them on a small patch of skin first.

43.   Take a warm bath to relieve eczema-related itching. Make sure that the water is lukewarm. Consider using a bit of colloidal oatmeal or baking soda for a soothing bath. Bleach is even useful. Pour a small amount in a large bath, and it will help reduce the bacteria colonies that inhabit the skin.

44.   Try to avoid stress. Too much stress can trigger eczema. Of course, eczema is itchy and unpleasant and can lead to even more stress. Break the cycle by finding ways to unwind. Find a new, relaxing hobby. Devote a few days a week to getting some

exercise. Find a method of getting rid of stress that works for you.

45.   If you have any of the many types of eczema, you should keep your fingernails cut short. Although individuals try to refrain from scratching the patches of dry, itchy skin, sometimes scratching is done as a reflex without conscious though. With shortened nails, it's less likely that the dry, delicate skin will be punctured when you scratch it.

46.   Get in the bath if you feel an eczema break-out coming on. Not only does the bath add some much needed moisture to your skin, but it also is needed to remove debris and irritants that may be causing the break out. Don't add oils or perfumes to the bath.

47.   Moisturize your skin immediately after taking a bath. Applying lotion to your skin soon after your bath helps to lock in the moisture and prevents your skin from drying too much. For the best results, use a intensive moisturizer that does not have added perfumes or dyes, which can dry your skin more.

48.   Make good use of creams containing hydrocortisone. A 1% solution will help ease itching. You can use this type of preparation two or

three times a day for a week. Be careful not to overuse it because it is a steroid. Using it for too long could be unsafe.

49.   Take care not to scratch. If you tend to scratch in your sleep, be sure the itchy areas are covered by gauze, bandages or pajamas. Trim your fingernails very short so that you will not be able to scratch much while sleeping. Use cold compresses and/or anti-itch treatments right before bed.

50.   Have your doctor run some tests to identify any allergies you may have. It is possible your eczema is an allergic reaction to products like gluten, peanuts, soy or dairy. These are common allergens, and it's a good idea to avoid them. Add soothing substances like vitamin A and vitamin D, fish oils, coconut oil and fish oils to your diet.

51.   If you prescribed or preferred moisturized comes in a tub, do not use your hands to scoop it out. This puts bacteria in the moisturizer that can get into your blood stream during a breakout. Use a spoon or spatula to get enough moisturizer out of the tub to use. Make sure to clean the spoon between uses.

52.   As you may already know, when you have a flare-up with your eczema, the itching associated

with it is almost unbearable. You want to scratch the affected skin, but you know that if you do it will only make the situation worse. A cold compress can curb your desire to scratch. The compress provides some relief because it reduces inflammation of the affected skin cells.

53.   Avoid scratching your skin in areas that have eczema. This will only aid in making the skin itchier and will increase the inflammation. It could also cause infection. If you need to calm the itch, try applying a cooling gel or moisturizer. Make sure fingernails are clipped short, as well.

54.   If you are getting ready to put something on your skin to moisturize it, like an ointment or a lotion, make sure you get your skin damp first. That will help the moisturizer do its job. It may be best to apply the product within a few minutes of getting out the shower or the bath. Simply pat yourself dry, so that you are not dripping wet, and then put the product on.

55.   Know what your triggers are so you can avoid them. Your triggers may laundry detergent, soaps, and dust. You should probably steer clear of any products that contain fragrances, chemicals or other unnatural additives. Choose pure and unscented

products instead. This will help to reduce the discomfort of daily eczema flare-ups.

56.   If you have eczema, rubbing your skin with a towel to get it dry may aggravate your eczema and lead to a flare-up. Rubbing produces friction which can irritate sensitive skin areas. It also removes your body's naturals oils. When drying you body after bathing, use a towel to pat your skin until it's partially dry. While your skin is still a bit damp, apply a moisturizer to lock in the bath's moisture.

57.   Avoid becoming overheated. Excess sweat can trigger eczema flare-ups. If you do work out, take a shower afterwards. In fact, shower after any bout of strenuous activity, which could include things like gardening or heavy housework. Keeping your skin clean will help to keep you comfortable and your eczema flare-ups at bay.

58.   Do not scratch your eczema. It is hard to resist because eczema is an itchy skin condition, but scratching makes it worse. You can increase the itching, damage your skin, and increase your risk of getting an infection. Try keeping the skin moisturized, bathing regularly, and using cold compresses to alleviate itching.

59.   Moisturize immediately following bathing. This is the best time to do it because your skin is still damp. Make sure to only pat dry your skin between showering and moisturizing. You don't want to remove any moisture that your skin has already absorbed; that is counterproductive to treating your eczema.

60.   One common misconception about proper skin care of those who have eczema is to keep bathing to a minimum because it dries out the skin. Actually, dermatologists recommend that those who have atopic dermatitis should take a short, daily shower or bath in tepid water to hydrate their skin. However, it's important that the water is lukewarm and not hot.

61.   Keep your hands protected. These eczema-prone areas are exposed to water and irritating substances like cleaning products. Too much moisture or sweat can trigger symptoms. When you need to submerge them in water, try using rubber gloves. Wearing cotton gloves can also keep hands protected when doing work around the house. Try wearing cotton or leather gloves when doing outside work.

62.   Be wary of changes in temperature. A dramatic change in temperature can cause your eczema to

flare up. Try to keep your home a temperature that will not aggravate your skin. Be sure to use air conditioning when it is particularly hot out. When it is cold, use a humidifier to keep your skin from drying out.

63.   Never take extremely hot showers. Hot showers can irritate the skin. Limit your hot showers if you have eczema. Keep the water at room temperature when you shower. Gently clean skin with a gentle cleanser and moisturize after.

64.   Make sure to put gloves on your hands. It is vital that you protect your hands. When doing dishes, avoid irritating the skin by wearing rubber gloves. Cotton gloves work well if you are just doing a bit of housework. Leather gloves are nice for cold weather. Avoid wool whenever possible. This fabric can be quite irritating.

65.   Take care not to scratch. If you tend to scratch in your sleep, be sure the itchy areas are covered by gauze, bandages or pajamas. Trim your fingernails very short so that you will not be able to scratch much while sleeping. Use cold compresses and/or anti-itch treatments right before bed.

66.   You may already know to change your sheets frequently but have you considered your curtains?

Your curtains can attract a great amount of dust over time and that dust is released in the air whenever you open and close them. So you should wash them frequently or invest in some that are easier for you to wash.

67.	Remove tags from clothes and avoid rough seams. The seams and tags can scratch the skin, making eczema worse. Buy clothes with no tags in them or cut them out. Be watchful for seams that can cause discomfort through extended wear. If your seams are in your underwear, you may want to turn things inside out.

68.	One key factor in controlling eczema is to daily practice good skin care. When washing your skin, it's best to use a soap substitute or a mild soap. These cleansing agents are less likely to dry out your skin. Immediately after bathing, always apply a good moisturizer. Moisturizers help conserve your skin's natural moisture.

69.	Keep the temperature constant in your house. That means you will have to use your air conditioning system at different points throughout the year. If the temperature fluctuates too much, that can be a trigger for your eczema. During the winter, it may be best to get a cool mist humidifier as well, so that your skin does not dry out.

70.   Your body temperature could have an impact on your eczema. Being too hot could cause you to sweat, which makes the skin irritated and itchy. In the winter time, the humidity inside is quite low, which could cause the skin to dry out and become itchy. Keep these things in mind as to what could make your eczema flare up.

71.   Pay attention to your hands. Because you wash them throughout the day, they can get very dry and are prone to more eczema. If you are engaged in an activity that involves water, like washing the dishes, wear rubber gloves. This will help protect your skin from the water throughout the day.

72.   You should always use sunscreen. This is even more important when you have eczema. Use a sunscreen with an SPF of at least 30 so you don't get a sunburn. Having a sunburn can make your skin even itchier than usual. You could use sunscreens specifically formulated for the face on the entire body. These are generally more gentle to use.

73.   If you have been prescribed medicine for your eczema, take it as directed. When all else fails, your doctor may be able to help ease your symptoms by prescribing you something a little stronger than

what you can get over the counter. While no one really wants to rely on medication, sometimes it is necessary.

74.   Try to be aware of anything that triggers your eczema. Flare ups of eczema can be particularly unpleasant. It is important to know what makes your eczema worse. Do scented soaps or lotions aggravate your skin? Make note of anything that causes your eczema to flare up, and make a point to avoid it.

75.   Keep your hands protected. Wear rubber gloves while washing dishes or performing another activity in which your hands are submersed in water. For further protection, wear cotton gloves underneath the rubber ones to reduce sweat and irritation. Use the cotton gloves while performing other activities, such as gardening and housework.

76.   Get your skin damp before applying your moisturizer. This helps the moisturizer to seal into your skin and soften it. Following your shower or bath, just pat your skin with a towel. This will remove a lot of the wetness but still leave the skin damp and ready for moisturizing.

77.   One effective skin care regimen which will reduce flare-ups and improve response to

medication and treatment is proper application of moisturizers. Moisturizers trap moisture in the skin, so applying moisturizers no later than 3 minutes after bathing is highly effective. Of course, it is still important to continue to apply a moisturizer to very dry patches of skin throughout the day.

78.   If you live in an area that experiences cold weather in the winter, buy a humidifier to help decrease eczema flare-ups. During the cold winter months, we close all of our windows and turn on the furnace. This can make the air inside of a house very dry which makes the itching and dry skin associated with eczema even worse. To replace moisture in your internal environment, use a humidifier. This added moisture will keep your skin from becoming dry, cracked, itchy and irritated.

79.   Try to avoid stress. Too much stress can trigger eczema. Of course, eczema is itchy and unpleasant and can lead to even more stress. Break the cycle by finding ways to unwind. Find a new, relaxing hobby. Devote a few days a week to getting some exercise. Find a method of getting rid of stress that works for you.

80.   Moisturize your skin immediately after taking a bath. Applying lotion to your skin soon after your bath helps to lock in the moisture and prevents

your skin from drying too much. For the best results, use a intensive moisturizer that does not have added perfumes or dyes, which can dry your skin more.

81.   Take a bath at least once a day. Showers are great for getting clean, but sitting in the tub is the best way to soothe and moisturize your skin. You do not need to limit yourself to one bath a day. If you find that it helps, take as many baths as you need to.

82.   If you have eczema occasionally, an outbreak may be related to other things that cause allergies. Avoid using strong household chemicals as much as possible, as well as perfumed laundry products. Take care to notice if any type of pattern develops that may associate an outbreak with any of these products.

83.   When you buy new sheets, always wash them first. They may seem clean and fresh but they are likely stiff with starch or other chemicals that can be irritating to your skin. So give them a wash with a gentle detergent and use an unscented softener to reduce the risk of irritation to your skin.

84.   Lotions and creams do not usually work as well as ointments. Ointments have a bit more oil in

them, which generally helps them moisturize more effectively. They are a little harder to apply than creams, however, but they are much better at adding a protective layer to the skin and easing your symptoms.

85.   Be careful when you put on sunscreen. You never know what may cause you to have an outbreak of eczema. The higher the SPF, the more likely it is that the sunscreen may cause you to have an issue. Try and find something with an SPF of around 35. That should protect your skin from the sun and keep it in good shape overall.

86.   Resist the urge to scratch. Scratching will only intensify that itchy feeling. It can also cause harm to your skin, including infection. Find other ways to relieve that itch. Use moisturizers, medications, cold compresses, and long soaks in the tub instead. These methods relieve your itch and make you feel better.

87.   Winter weather can cause eczema to worsen. Anytime your skin is exposed to frigid air, it needs a protective barrier to protect it from moisture loss. On any skin areas, such as the face or neck, be sure to heavily apply a moisturizer. Moisturizers will help you avoid dry and cracking skin because it locks in your skin's natural oils.

88.   Keep your hands protected. Wear rubber gloves while washing dishes or performing another activity in which your hands are submersed in water. For further protection, wear cotton gloves underneath the rubber ones to reduce sweat and irritation. Use the cotton gloves while performing other activities, such as gardening and housework.

89.   So, you think you have eczema. Have you visited a doctor yet to confirm your self-diagnosis? Not only are there several kinds of eczema, there are also several skin condition which are quite similar to eczema. Only a professional, such as a dermatologist has the education and experience to make an accurate diagnosis. The only way to experience effective treatment is by having an accurate diagnosis of your condition.

90.   For those that have eczema, skin care must be modified in the cold, dry winter months. During these months, you should use an oil-based moisturizer. The oil in these moisturizers promote moisture retention. The best form of moisturizer to use in these circumstances is an ointment due to the amount of oil it contains. Since ointments are 80% oil, it protects the skin more effectively than either lotions or creams.

91.	If you live in an area that experiences cold weather in the winter, buy a humidifier to help decrease eczema flare-ups. During the cold winter months, we close all of our windows and turn on the furnace. This can make the air inside of a house very dry which makes the itching and dry skin associated with eczema even worse. To replace moisture in your internal environment, use a humidifier. This added moisture will keep your skin from becoming dry, cracked, itchy and irritated.

92.	Try to avoid over-bathing. Too much water irritates eczema. Spending more than 10 minutes in direct water stops moisturizing the skin. It actually dries it out. If you are unable to bathe within 5 to 10 minutes, try streamlining your bathing routine to make it as short and thorough as possible.

93.	People that have eczema are prone to skin infections. When the skin is irritated, sometimes its surface cracks and gaps are formed. Germs can envade the skin through these gaps and cause an infection. To reduce this risk, use a mild, non-drying cleanser on your skin to remove dirt, bacteria, and other foreign matter. Gently apply the cleanser with your fingertips and rinse it off with tepid water.

94.   Talk to your doctor. Eczema is unpleasant, and you shouldn't have to suffer because of it. Get some professional advice if managing your eczema proves too difficult. A doctor can usually help determine what is causing your eczema, give you advice, and prescribe something to help, like a cream or antihistamine.

95.   Moisturize your skin immediately after taking a bath. Applying lotion to your skin soon after your bath helps to lock in the moisture and prevents your skin from drying too much. For the best results, use a intensive moisturizer that does not have added perfumes or dyes, which can dry your skin more.

96.   Consider getting rid of your carpets and throw rugs throughout your house. Carpet and rugs are known for harboring dust mites, allergens and other microscopic irritants which can cause an eczema flair-up. So consider hardwood floors or a low pile carpet if you absolutely must have carpet in your house.

97.   If you have eczema occasionally, an outbreak may be related to other things that cause allergies. Avoid using strong household chemicals as much as possible, as well as perfumed laundry products. Take care to notice if any type of pattern develops

that may associate an outbreak with any of these products.

98.   Have your doctor run some tests to identify any allergies you may have. It is possible your eczema is an allergic reaction to products like gluten, peanuts, soy or dairy. These are common allergens, and it's a good idea to avoid them. Add soothing substances like vitamin A and vitamin D, fish oils, coconut oil and fish oils to your diet.

99.   Some individuals that have a severe case of eczema find relief by taking their baths in water which has a small portion of bleach added to it. This helps because the bleach actually kills bacteria which takes up residence on the skin of those who are plagued with eczema. Of course, don't take a long bath or use really hot water because both can rob your skin of its natural moisture.

100.   As you may already know, when you have a flare-up with your eczema, the itching associated with it is almost unbearable. You want to scratch the affected skin, but you know that if you do it will only make the situation worse. A cold compress can curb your desire to scratch. The compress provides some relief because it reduces inflammation of the affected skin cells.

101.   Keep the temperature constant in your house. That means you will have to use your air conditioning system at different points throughout the year. If the temperature fluctuates too much, that can be a trigger for your eczema. During the winter, it may be best to get a cool mist humidifier as well, so that your skin does not dry out.

102.   You should always use sunscreen. This is even more important when you have eczema. Use a sunscreen with an SPF of at least 30 so you don't get a sunburn. Having a sunburn can make your skin even itchier than usual. You could use sunscreens specifically formulated for the face on the entire body. These are generally more gentle to use.

103.   There are several medications you can try to help relieve the itching of eczema. Topical treatments including calamine lotion, which helps soothe the itching. Another topical option is an over-the-counter cream that contains one percent hydrocortisone. For severe itching, consider an oral over-the-counter antihistamine, such as Benadryl. Follow the instructions on the package, and remember that antihistamines may cause drowsiness.

104.   Control your indoor temperature. Eczema tends to flare up during shifts in temps or humidity. Use your air conditioner to stay cool in the warmer months. A humidifier can help you keep your skin from drying out during colder weather. Staying comfortable temp wise will help reduce the frequency of flare ups.

105.   If you have eczema, rubbing your skin with a towel to get it dry may aggravate your eczema and lead to a flare-up. Rubbing produces friction which can irritate sensitive skin areas. It also removes your body's naturals oils. When drying you body after bathing, use a towel to pat your skin until it's partially dry. While your skin is still a bit damp, apply a moisturizer to lock in the bath's moisture.

106.   If you have eczema, you should moisturize your skin regularly. This is a great way to manage your flare-ups. Keep your skin well hydrated by moisturizing after baths or showers. Try to use plain moisturizers that are fragrance-free and that do not contain harsh chemicals or additives.

107.   Do not scratch your eczema. It is hard to resist because eczema is an itchy skin condition, but scratching makes it worse. You can increase the itching, damage your skin, and increase your risk of getting an infection. Try keeping the skin

moisturized, bathing regularly, and using cold compresses to alleviate itching.

108.   For those that have eczema, skin care must be modified in the cold, dry winter months. During these months, you should use an oil-based moisturizer. The oil in these moisturizers promote moisture retention. The best form of moisturizer to use in these circumstances is an ointment due to the amount of oil it contains. Since ointments are 80% oil, it protects the skin more effectively than either lotions or creams.

109.   Sweeping can cause issues with dust, and dust is not good for eczema. Vacuuming will keep the house clean while helping you to avoid flare-ups. While you have the cleaner out, head up to the bedrooms and vacuum the mattresses as well. This will help ensure that your room stays as dust-free as possible.

110.   Be wary of changes in temperature. A dramatic change in temperature can cause your eczema to flare up. Try to keep your home a temperature that will not aggravate your skin. Be sure to use air conditioning when it is particularly hot out. When it is cold, use a humidifier to keep your skin from drying out.

111.   Never scratch at itchy skin. Eczema can be quite itchy and unpleasant. It is important that you avoid the temptation to scratch. Scratching can cause your skin to only itch more. Worse, it could lead to infection. Find other ways to manage your itching. Try using medications or cold compresses.

112.   Should your eczema start to bother you, do not itch, no matter how tempted you are to do so. Scratching not only makes itching worse, but it can actually irritate your skin and even cause infection. Try to find other ways to deal with the itching; apply cold compresses to the affected area or use medications.

113.   Moisturize your skin immediately after taking a bath. Applying lotion to your skin soon after your bath helps to lock in the moisture and prevents your skin from drying too much. For the best results, use a intensive moisturizer that does not have added perfumes or dyes, which can dry your skin more.

114.   If you have an occasional eczema outbreak, it may caused by things that also cause allergies. Avoid things like harsh household detergents and scented laundry products. Pay attention to whether or not you have had a reaction to any types of products.

115.   Manage your stress. If you are upset, your eczema may flare up, which will only exacerbate an already frustrating situation. Learn how to deal with stress and keep yourself from getting too wound up. For example, deep breathing is one thing you can do just about anywhere to help keep your stress levels down.

116.   If you are getting ready to put something on your skin to moisturize it, like an ointment or a lotion, make sure you get your skin damp first. That will help the moisturizer do its job. It may be best to apply the product within a few minutes of getting out the shower or the bath. Simply pat yourself dry, so that you are not dripping wet, and then put the product on.

117.   Know what your triggers are so you can avoid them. Your triggers may laundry detergent, soaps, and dust. You should probably steer clear of any products that contain fragrances, chemicals or other unnatural additives. Choose pure and unscented products instead. This will help to reduce the discomfort of daily eczema flare-ups.

118.   Do not scratch your eczema. It is hard to resist because eczema is an itchy skin condition, but scratching makes it worse. You can increase the itching, damage your skin, and increase your risk of

getting an infection. Try keeping the skin moisturized, bathing regularly, and using cold compresses to alleviate itching.

119.   Eczema can make a person have itchy and dry skin. To reduce these symptoms apply a moisturizer often. Moisturizers don't hydrate your skin. Actually, frequently applying moisturizers helps lock in a person's natural body oils and moisture. This will reduce the amount of dryness that you have.

120.   One effective skin care regimen which will reduce flare-ups and improve response to medication and treatment is proper application of moisturizers. Moisturizers trap moisture in the skin, so applying moisturizers no later than 3 minutes after bathing is highly effective. Of course, it is still important to continue to apply a moisturizer to very dry patches of skin throughout the day.

121.   Don't take too many hot showers. While they can feel good, they tend to irritate the skin tremendously. If you struggle with eczema, limit how many hot showers that you take. Rather, look to getting showers with room temperature water. Use a gentle, cotton cloth to clean the skin an apply a moisturizer after you are done.

122.   Eczema is a skin condition that produces red, itchy, dry and cracked skin. Using moisturizer frequently will help treat the symptoms and provide some relief. Petroleum jelly is an excellent moisturizer that contains no perfumes to irritate the skin. Keep a jar of petroleum jelly near every sink and use it throughout the day to soothe and add moisture to your skin.

123.   Moisturize your skin immediately after taking a bath. Applying lotion to your skin soon after your bath helps to lock in the moisture and prevents your skin from drying too much. For the best results, use a intensive moisturizer that does not have added perfumes or dyes, which can dry your skin more.

124.   It is important to avoid too much stress if you suffer from eczema. Of course, having the skin condition can cause stress, as can life itself. But, a lot of stress increases flare-ups. If you find yourself getting stressed out, learn how to relax yourself. Yoga and meditation are two great ideas.

125.   Instead of scratching, try using ice to cool itchy areas. You can get an inexpensive gel compress and keep it in the freezer. Take it out and hold it over itchy areas whenever you need to. Keep a dry washcloth in your purse or pocket at all times. If

you become very itchy away from home, soak the cloth in cold water. Hold it over the itchy area.

126. During the summer months, beware of which sunscreens you use if you have eczema. Every eczema sufferer has certain triggers, but sunscreen lotions are a common one. If you try multiple sunscreens and every one of them seem to cause a flare-up, you may want to chat with your doctor about a prescription alternative.

127. Always preform a patch test. When you are trying a new product, it is important to know whether or not it will irritate your skin before putting it all over yourself. Take a small amount of the product and apply it to a small portion of your skin. After a few hours, you should be able to determine whether or not it triggers your eczema.

128. You may think that keeping your house tightly sealed with help keep the dust and allergens down. But in fact it just traps them and allows them to accumulate. It is better to have ventilation in your house and to use a good heap filter where needed to capture the offending particles.

129. Vacuuming is a better choice than sweeping. Sweeping will stir up the dust and put it back into the air. Using a vacuum (with a good filtering bag)

will capture the particles and remove them from the air you breathe and keep them from resettling on the surfaces of your house.

130.   When you buy new sheets, always wash them first. They may seem clean and fresh but they are likely stiff with starch or other chemicals that can be irritating to your skin. So give them a wash with a gentle detergent and use an unscented softener to reduce the risk of irritation to your skin.

131.   Do not take a hot shower if you are dealing with eczema. Your showers you take daily should be short and warm. Steer clear of soaps and choose gentle cleansers. Pat your skin to dry it.

132.   Avoid scratching your skin in areas that have eczema. This will only aid in making the skin itchier and will increase the inflammation. It could also cause infection. If you need to calm the itch, try applying a cooling gel or moisturizer. Make sure fingernails are clipped short, as well.

133.   Be careful when you put on sunscreen. You never know what may cause you to have an outbreak of eczema. The higher the SPF, the more likely it is that the sunscreen may cause you to have an issue. Try and find something with an SPF of

around 35. That should protect your skin from the sun and keep it in good shape overall.

134.   Resist the urge to scratch. Scratching will only intensify that itchy feeling. It can also cause harm to your skin, including infection. Find other ways to relieve that itch. Use moisturizers, medications, cold compresses, and long soaks in the tub instead. These methods relieve your itch and make you feel better.

135.   One effective skin care regimen which will reduce flare-ups and improve response to medication and treatment is proper application of moisturizers. Moisturizers trap moisture in the skin, so applying moisturizers no later than 3 minutes after bathing is highly effective. Of course, it is still important to continue to apply a moisturizer to very dry patches of skin throughout the day.

136.   Try to avoid over-bathing. Too much water irritates eczema. Spending more than 10 minutes in direct water stops moisturizing the skin. It actually dries it out. If you are unable to bathe within 5 to 10 minutes, try streamlining your bathing routine to make it as short and thorough as possible.

137.   Studies have shown that setting a text message as a reminder can be effective in treating atopic

dermatitis. This skin condition is common for anyone suffering with eczema. Text messages work for patients 14 and older. This helps people stick to a regimen and lessens eczema. Many patients were desirous of continuing to get the messages.

138.   If you have eczema, you should apply moisturizer while the skin is damp. This will help your skin retain the most moisture throughout the day. First, blot the skin with a towel to keep it moist and help it retain natural oils. Next, use your moisturizing product. This should be a process that takes just a few minutes after bath time.

139.   Talk to your doctor. Eczema is unpleasant, and you shouldn't have to suffer because of it. Get some professional advice if managing your eczema proves too difficult. A doctor can usually help determine what is causing your eczema, give you advice, and prescribe something to help, like a cream or antihistamine.

140.   It is important to avoid too much stress if you suffer from eczema. Of course, having the skin condition can cause stress, as can life itself. But, a lot of stress increases flare-ups. If you find yourself getting stressed out, learn how to relax yourself. Yoga and meditation are two great ideas.

141.   Buy a good humidifier and use it when the air is dry. You might use if year round in a dry, arid climate. If you live in a humid climate, you might only need to use it in the winter when your heater is on, pumping out dry, hot air which quickly dries out skin.

142.   Eczema outbreaks may be caused by allergens. Keep the use of chemicals down in the house, and steer clear of anything perfumed, like detergents and creams. Focus on the effects of chemicals so you can eliminate any that trigger flare-ups.

143.   If you have eczema occasionally, an outbreak may be related to other things that cause allergies. Avoid using strong household chemicals as much as possible, as well as perfumed laundry products. Take care to notice if any type of pattern develops that may associate an outbreak with any of these products.

144.   Have your doctor run some tests to identify any allergies you may have. It is possible your eczema is an allergic reaction to products like gluten, peanuts, soy or dairy. These are common allergens, and it's a good idea to avoid them. Add soothing substances like vitamin A and vitamin D, fish oils, coconut oil and fish oils to your diet.

145.   Avoid feather pillows and opt for a pillow that is less likely to attract and keep dust mites. Foam pillows may be a better choice for you and you can also invest in pillowcases that help keep dust, dust mites and allergens from getting into the pillow in the first place.

146.   Avoid carpeting, if you can. Much like people who suffer from allergies, eczema sufferers can face issues with carpeting and rugs. These items retain a lot of dirt and dust which trigger flare-ups. It's best to stick with hard flooring like wood and tile.

147.   Certain foods you eat can cause your eczema to flare up. However, it is sometimes hard to figure out which foods are causing your flare-ups. Therefore, it is a good idea to keep a food diary. Document each food you consume each day so you can find a pattern of which foods cause flare-ups.

148.   No doubt extreme weather in both directions and consistent fluctuation between the two can cause you to have eczema flareups. However, while you can't do a thing about the conditions outside, you certainly can make sure you do what is necessary within your home. During those hot days, keep you air conditioning system going so that your skin stays moist, and an cool mist humidifier is perfect for the winter months.

149.   Your body temperature could have an impact on your eczema. Being too hot could cause you to sweat, which makes the skin irritated and itchy. In the winter time, the humidity inside is quite low, which could cause the skin to dry out and become itchy. Keep these things in mind as to what could make your eczema flare up.

150.   Try to be aware of anything that triggers your eczema. Flare ups of eczema can be particularly unpleasant. It is important to know what makes your eczema worse. Do scented soaps or lotions aggravate your skin? Make note of anything that causes your eczema to flare up, and make a point to avoid it.

151.   If you are dealing with eczema, then it is very important that your skin is moisturized properly each day. When it comes to controlling flareups, this is among the best ways. Use moisturizers as often as possible. The best time to use them is directly after a show or bath. Stick to unscented products that are low on chemicals and added ingredients.

152.   Do not scratch your eczema. It is hard to resist because eczema is an itchy skin condition, but scratching makes it worse. You can increase the

itching, damage your skin, and increase your risk of getting an infection. Try keeping the skin moisturized, bathing regularly, and using cold compresses to alleviate itching.

153.   Always make sure your fingernails are clean and short. You know during the day to avoid scratching your eczema, but you might do it anyway when you sleep. Short nails will reduce the irritation that you experience. Make sure you're cleaning under the nails on a regular basis.

154.   Remember to moisturize your skin. Moisturizing your skin regularly is one of the best ways you can combat eczema. Look for thick, unscented moisturizers that will not aggravate your skin. Too many chemicals or additives in a moisturizer can be counterproductive. Apply it on a daily basis, especially after taking a shower or bath.

155.   Find the triggers for your eczema. Could it be dust mites? Others may have issues with scented soaps. No matter the trigger, once you know, you can take steps to improve your life. This may involve a change in your daily habits, however if it means not having to deal with your eczema, it is worth the trouble.

156.   The exact cause of eczema is a mystery, and no cure exists. However, treatments that work are out there. Dry cracked skin on your hands is called dishpan hands, a type of eczema. Try to use gloves when you are doing the dishes. If you've got a latex-sensitivity, try wearing thin cotton gloves underneath for keeping your skin protected. When you are finished washing the dishes, use moisturizer.

157.   Make sure you wear gloves. This will help protect your hands. If you are washing dishes, wearing rubber gloves can help. When you do chores, wear cotton gloves, and wear leather gloves in the cold. Wool will irritate the skin so avoid this if you can. Wool can make it to where your skin gets irritated.

158.   You might be allergic to something which is causing your eczema. Steer clear of excessively strong household cleaners and heavily perfumed detergents. Do you see anything being a trigger for your outbreaks?

159.   Always wash your bedding, blankets and pillows on a regular basis. Don't wait until they seem dirty. Do it at least once a week to keep you bed as free from allergens and irritants as possible. Use a gentle detergent and softener that doesn't contain harsh

chemicals or fragrances which can cause irritation to sensitive people.

160.   Keep your nails clean and trimmed. Itching from eczema is to be expected. However, if you have long, dirty nails, itching your skin can cause an infection. Avoid that circumstance by trimming your nails and cleaning them.

161.   If you are taking a bath, using bath oil or scented beads that contain oils are a great way to help soothe dry and scratchy skin. Your skin will absorb the moisture from the bath and the oils will help your skin to retain that moisture and protect your skin from drying out.

162.   Only wear soft, comfortable, natural materials. Don't wear clothes that are scratchy, itchy or irritating in any way. Organic cotton is an excellent choice in clothing materials for people with eczema. Always be sure to wash your new clothing items before you wear them. This will remove preservatives and any other chemicals that might be on the cloth.

163.   You have likely been told to avoid the sun if you suffer from eczema. It's true that an abundance of sun can burn your skin. But know that Vitamin D deficiency is also a key component of eczema

breakouts. This is caused from not enough sun exposure. Make sure you do get some sun, about 15 minutes daily would do it.

164.   Always vacuum instead of sweeping. Sweeping just sweeps dirt, dust and other irritants into the air. This can irritate your skin and make your eczema worse. If you do not have carpeting in your home purchase a vacuum that you can use on hardwood floors as well. The investment will be worth it.

165.   Understand what makes your eczema act up. It could be that there is a certain type of soap that gets you every time, for example. In most cases, you do not want to use anything that has a scent attached to it. That means it may be necessary to avoid perfume, some body lotions and even certain types of make-up.

166.   Keep the temperature constant in your house. That means you will have to use your air conditioning system at different points throughout the year. If the temperature fluctuates too much, that can be a trigger for your eczema. During the winter, it may be best to get a cool mist humidifier as well, so that your skin does not dry out.

167.   Lotions and creams do not usually work as well as ointments. Ointments have a bit more oil in

them, which generally helps them moisturize more effectively. They are a little harder to apply than creams, however, but they are much better at adding a protective layer to the skin and easing your symptoms.

168.   Resist the urge to scratch. Scratching will only intensify that itchy feeling. It can also cause harm to your skin, including infection. Find other ways to relieve that itch. Use moisturizers, medications, cold compresses, and long soaks in the tub instead. These methods relieve your itch and make you feel better.

169.   Be sure that the clothes you wear do not cause skin irritation. There are certain fabrics that if worn can actually cause eczema flareups. Cotton is the best choice in fabrics to wear. Also, wash all new clothes before you ever wear them. Mild detergent that is unscented should be used and never use softener.

170.   Moisturize your skin if you have eczema. This is one of the best ways to keep your flare-ups under control. Make sure that you moisturize each and every day. Don't use any moisturizers that contain alcohols or scents because they will irritate the skin.

171.   So, you think you have eczema. Have you visited a doctor yet to confirm your self-diagnosis? Not only are there several kinds of eczema, there are also several skin condition which are quite similar to eczema. Only a professional, such as a dermatologist has the education and experience to make an accurate diagnosis. The only way to experience effective treatment is by having an accurate diagnosis of your condition.

172.   Remember to moisturize your skin. Moisturizing your skin regularly is one of the best ways you can combat eczema. Look for thick, unscented moisturizers that will not aggravate your skin. Too many chemicals or additives in a moisturizer can be counterproductive. Apply it on a daily basis, especially after taking a shower or bath.

173.   If you live in an area that experiences cold weather in the winter, buy a humidifier to help decrease eczema flare-ups. During the cold winter months, we close all of our windows and turn on the furnace. This can make the air inside of a house very dry which makes the itching and dry skin associated with eczema even worse. To replace moisture in your internal environment, use a humidifier. This added moisture will keep your skin from becoming dry, cracked, itchy and irritated.

174.   There are specific eczema triggers, plenty of
them, and you need to realize what they are. Soaps,
perfumes, detergents and other scented items could
be causing your eczema. Stress and sweat are two
other factors that should be considered as possible
triggers. When you pinpoint what your triggers are,
make sure that you avoid these things as much as
possible.

175.   Most patients with eczema already know how
important it is to moisturize their skin. But, what
many do not know is the proper way to moisturize
it. For starters, use a product that is unscented and
contains no chemicals, as this can bother your skin.
Also, be sure to moisturize frequently, especially
after you shower.

176.   Take a bath at least once a day. Showers are
great for getting clean, but sitting in the tub is the
best way to soothe and moisturize your skin. You
do not need to limit yourself to one bath a day. If
you find that it helps, take as many baths as you
need to.

177.   If you have eczema occasionally, an outbreak
may be related to other things that cause allergies.
Avoid using strong household chemicals as much as
possible, as well as perfumed laundry products.
Take care to notice if any type of pattern develops

that may associate an outbreak with any of these products.

178.   When taking a bath, don't use excessively hot water. It will dry out your skin which will aggravate your eczema. Use warm water, a gentle soap and a soft rag to clean any patches of eczema that you have. If you really want to use a loofah or a scrubbie then only use it on unaffected areas and rinse, clean and dry the loofah or scrubbie afterwards.

179.   Find out if you are allergic to anything in your immediate environment. If you are allergic, take steps to remove the allergen or mitigate exposure to it. Build up your immune system with B and C vitamins and a healthy diet. This will reduce any allergic reactions you may experience.

180.   Avoid too many dairy products if you have eczema. The milk from a cow contains hormones and chemicals that lower the immune system and cause flareups. While having dairy products occasionally is fine, do not go overboard; there are many great, tasty substitutes to many dairy products, like almond milk and goat milk.

181.   Make your moisturizer your best friend. Every time you wash your hands or take a bath, apply the

moisturizer. Do not get fancy. Anything that has a scent attached to it could exacerbate your condition. Also, look for a very thick product to get the best results for your skin.

182.   If you have been prescribed medicine for your eczema, take it as directed. When all else fails, your doctor may be able to help ease your symptoms by prescribing you something a little stronger than what you can get over the counter. While no one really wants to rely on medication, sometimes it is necessary.

183.   There are several medications you can try to help relieve the itching of eczema. Topical treatments including calamine lotion, which helps soothe the itching. Another topical option is an over-the-counter cream that contains one percent hydrocortisone. For severe itching, consider an oral over-the-counter antihistamine, such as Benadryl. Follow the instructions on the package, and remember that antihistamines may cause drowsiness.

184.   Winter weather can cause eczema to worsen. Anytime your skin is exposed to frigid air, it needs a protective barrier to protect it from moisture loss. On any skin areas, such as the face or neck, be sure to heavily apply a moisturizer. Moisturizers will help

you avoid dry and cracking skin because it locks in your skin's natural oils.

185.   Get your skin damp before applying your moisturizer. This helps the moisturizer to seal into your skin and soften it. Following your shower or bath, just pat your skin with a towel. This will remove a lot of the wetness but still leave the skin damp and ready for moisturizing.

186.   Experiment with suntan lotions to find one that works for you. Certain sunscreens may exacerbate your eczema while others will not. However, what works for one person doesn't necessarily work for another. Keep trying them until you find one you can live with. However, be sure to just test them on a small patch of skin first.

187.   Use an antibiotic ointment on severely cracked skin. This can prevent infections from forming. It also serves as a moisturizer. Do this sparingly though; prolonged use of antibiotic ointments can render them ineffective. If you do have an infection, you should consult your doctor, who may give you an oral antibiotic.

188.   One common misconception about proper skin care of those who have eczema is to keep bathing to a minimum because it dries out the skin.

Actually, dermatologists recommend that those who have atopic dermatitis should take a short, daily shower or bath in tepid water to hydrate their skin. However, it's important that the water is lukewarm and not hot.

189.   Keep your stress levels down if you have eczema. The chances of having it flare up increase when you are stressed out. Stress can also make eczema itchier and more uncomfortable. That can create a never-ending cycle of anger and frustration from dealing with both your stress and your skin. Try relaxing by doing activities like yoga, deep breathing, and meditation.

190.   Speak with your doctor about your eczema if changing your lifestyle isn't enough. They may be able to help you find a medication that helps ease the symptoms. These medications can be over-the-counter antihistamines or creams. More serious cases may require a prescription medication. Make sure that whatever they suggest or give you is used as directed.

191.   Be wary of changes in temperature. A dramatic change in temperature can cause your eczema to flare up. Try to keep your home a temperature that will not aggravate your skin. Be sure to use air conditioning when it is particularly hot out. When it

is cold, use a humidifier to keep your skin from drying out.

192.   If you live in an area that experiences cold weather in the winter, buy a humidifier to help decrease eczema flare-ups. During the cold winter months, we close all of our windows and turn on the furnace. This can make the air inside of a house very dry which makes the itching and dry skin associated with eczema even worse. To replace moisture in your internal environment, use a humidifier. This added moisture will keep your skin from becoming dry, cracked, itchy and irritated.

193.   Most patients with eczema already know how important it is to moisturize their skin. But, what many do not know is the proper way to moisturize it. For starters, use a product that is unscented and contains no chemicals, as this can bother your skin. Also, be sure to moisturize frequently, especially after you shower.

194.   Make good use of creams containing hydrocortisone. A 1% solution will help ease itching. You can use this type of preparation two or three times a day for a week. Be careful not to overuse it because it is a steroid. Using it for too long could be unsafe.

195.   Buy a good humidifier and use it when the air is dry. You might use if year round in a dry, arid climate. If you live in a humid climate, you might only need to use it in the winter when your heater is on, pumping out dry, hot air which quickly dries out skin.

196.   If you have to use rubber or latex gloves, put on a pair of thin cotton gloves before you put the rubber or latex gloves on. This will help avoid a reaction to the rubber or latex and will help keep your hands protected from the sweat that these gloves can cause.

197.   Avoid hot showers. The water in any showers you take should be warm. The showers should be brief. Avoid using soap, rather use a gentle type of cleanser and avoid rubbing your skin while using it. Once your skin is clean, gently pat dry.

198.   When you have eczema, you should take caution to clean the skin gently. Once you have washed your skin, and it is still moist, apply a good moisturizer to the skin within three minutes to ensure the moisture is sealed into the skin. You may even want to soak in a nice oatmeal bath as well before you moisturize.

199.   Make your moisturizer your best friend. Every time you wash your hands or take a bath, apply the moisturizer. Do not get fancy. Anything that has a scent attached to it could exacerbate your condition. Also, look for a very thick product to get the best results for your skin.

200.   When buying a detergent, look for something that is not scented. If you are having trouble finding one that works for you, look for products labeled "free and clear" and see if they work. In addition, it may be best not to use a fabric softener at all. This product can cause an issue for people with eczema, so it is usually not worth the risk.

201.   Do not turn the water up too high when in the shower or the bath. It can cause problems for your eczema. In addition, be gentle when washing your skin. Do not rub the skin too hard, and avoid soap. Instead, use a cleanser that is safer for your body.

202.   You should always use sunscreen. This is even more important when you have eczema. Use a sunscreen with an SPF of at least 30 so you don't get a sunburn. Having a sunburn can make your skin even itchier than usual. You could use sunscreens specifically formulated for the face on the entire body. These are generally more gentle to use.

203. If you have been prescribed medicine for your eczema, take it as directed. When all else fails, your doctor may be able to help ease your symptoms by prescribing you something a little stronger than what you can get over the counter. While no one really wants to rely on medication, sometimes it is necessary.

204. Be careful when you put on sunscreen. You never know what may cause you to have an outbreak of eczema. The higher the SPF, the more likely it is that the sunscreen may cause you to have an issue. Try and find something with an SPF of around 35. That should protect your skin from the sun and keep it in good shape overall.

205. If you have eczema, rubbing your skin with a towel to get it dry may aggravate your eczema and lead to a flare-up. Rubbing produces friction which can irritate sensitive skin areas. It also removes your body's naturals oils. When drying you body after bathing, use a towel to pat your skin until it's partially dry. While your skin is still a bit damp, apply a moisturizer to lock in the bath's moisture.

206. Keep skin properly moisturized if you are afflicted with eczema. You will find this most effective in reducing flare-ups. Keep your skin

moisturized often after you bathe or shower to keep skin soft and pliable. Don't use any moisturizers that contain alcohols or scents because they will irritate the skin.

207.   Do not scratch your eczema. It is hard to resist because eczema is an itchy skin condition, but scratching makes it worse. You can increase the itching, damage your skin, and increase your risk of getting an infection. Try keeping the skin moisturized, bathing regularly, and using cold compresses to alleviate itching.

208.   So, you think you have eczema. Have you visited a doctor yet to confirm your self-diagnosis? Not only are there several kinds of eczema, there are also several skin condition which are quite similar to eczema. Only a professional, such as a dermatologist has the education and experience to make an accurate diagnosis. The only way to experience effective treatment is by having an accurate diagnosis of your condition.

209.   Don't cut off all exposure to the sun. Your eczema could be a result of a Vitamin D deficiency, so blocking out the sun entirely is not a good idea. You should be getting at least 10 to 15 minutes of sunlight a day sans sunscreen. Don't get any more than that though or you could burn.

210.   Studies have revealed that the use of text message reminders actually helps as a great tool for dealing with dermatitis. One of the most common forms of eczema is atopic dermatitis. Harvard researchers have shown that text messages are great for facilitating proper treatment in sufferers of at least 14 years of age. This method helped patients adhere to their treatments, which resulted in less eczema after 6 weeks. Many of these same patients chose to stick with text messages permanently.

211.   Use a humidifier for patchy eczema. Humidifiers puts moisture in the air. This creates a moist environment because the steam contains droplets of water. That way, your skin can stay comfortable and smooth regardless of the weather. Just keep your skin clean so you don't have other issues.

212.   It is important to avoid too much stress if you suffer from eczema. Of course, having the skin condition can cause stress, as can life itself. But, a lot of stress increases flare-ups. If you find yourself getting stressed out, learn how to relax yourself. Yoga and meditation are two great ideas.

213.   To help soothe dry, itchy skin that comes from eczema, opt for moisturizers in ointment or cream forms. These are better than lotions. You may even

just want to use petroleum jelly as a moisturizer. Whatever you're going to use, just be sure you get it alcohol free and fragrance free. Try to get your skin moisturized twice a day at least.

214.   If you have allergies, being exposed to what you are allergic to may make your eczema worse. Eczema is not an allergy, but some common allergens that could trigger eczema are dairy products, eggs, wheat and tomatoes. Other things that could make your eczema flare up are pet dander, pollen, dust and mold.

215.   Common treatments for eczema include topical creams and ointments that contain cortisone. You could try hydrocortisone that can be purchased at your local drug store. If this doesn't soothe your eczema, you should talk with your doctor about possibly getting a stronger prescription from him. These will work like other steroid creams, but will be able to be used for a longer time.

216.   When buying a detergent, look for something that is not scented. If you are having trouble finding one that works for you, look for products labeled "free and clear" and see if they work. In addition, it may be best not to use a fabric softener at all. This product can cause an issue for people with eczema, so it is usually not worth the risk.

217.   Try to be aware of anything that triggers your eczema. Flare ups of eczema can be particularly unpleasant. It is important to know what makes your eczema worse. Do scented soaps or lotions aggravate your skin? Make note of anything that causes your eczema to flare up, and make a point to avoid it.

218.   Avoid becoming overheated. Excess sweat can trigger eczema flare-ups. If you do work out, take a shower afterwards. In fact, shower after any bout of strenuous activity, which could include things like gardening or heavy housework. Keeping your skin clean will help to keep you comfortable and your eczema flare-ups at bay.

219.   There are several things you can do to keep yourself from scratching your eczema. The best thing to do is keep it covered. Loose clothing may work, or try bandages or dressings on the afflicted area. Keep your fingernails trimmed short, and consider wearing gloves when you go to bed to avoid scratching while you are sleeping.

220.   Keep your home's temperature comfortable. Temperatures that are too extreme can do a number on your skin and will make symptoms appear. Use the air conditioner when it is hot outside, and use a

humidifier when it's cold outside. Humid air prevents your skin from getting too dry.

221.   To reduce eczema flare-ups, there are some basic bathing rules you can follow. Use room temperature water in your tub or shower. Hot water can cause eczema flare-ups. Don't scrub your skin. Use a gentle soap alternative instead of soap itself. Pat your skin dry, and liberally apply moisturizer when you are done bathing.

222.   Dust can cause issues. Rather than dry dusting, use a damp dust method instead. This will help capture the dust, rather than simply spreading it around the home. Also, because rugs and carpets are a beacon for dust, try not to have them in the house if at all possible.

223.   If your baby has eczema, bathe him or her every day. This will help to keep the skin moisturized and free from infection. Besides hydrating your baby's skin to help keep flare-ups at bay, baths can be fun for babies, and you can use them as an opportunity to further bond with yours.

224.   Sweeping can cause issues with dust, and dust is not good for eczema. Vacuuming will keep the house clean while helping you to avoid flare-ups. While you have the cleaner out, head up to the

bedrooms and vacuum the mattresses as well. This will help ensure that your room stays as dust-free as possible.

225.   If your doctor has approved over-the-counter ointments for your eczema, make sure you get the right kinds. You should be looking at products that are only 20% water and 80% oil. While they may feel greasier, they will lock moisture in your skin better. Try not to use these products in areas that get sweaty.

226.   If you have any of the many types of eczema, you should keep your fingernails cut short. Although individuals try to refrain from scratching the patches of dry, itchy skin, sometimes scratching is done as a reflex without conscious though. With shortened nails, it's less likely that the dry, delicate skin will be punctured when you scratch it.

227.   When taking a bath or shower, use only very gentle cleansers. Don't scrub too hard. After you take a shower or a bath, pat your skin dry gently. Be sure to moisturize all over with a natural oil such as olive oil. This will help keep the moisture from your bath in your skin.

228.   The cause of eczema is not known, but certain people who also have allergies seem to be more

susceptible to the condition. They may have an outbreak due to stress, scratchy materials next to their skin or getting overheated. Many people are able to control the condition by avoiding these conditions.

229.   Do not turn the water up too high when in the shower or the bath. It can cause problems for your eczema. In addition, be gentle when washing your skin. Do not rub the skin too hard, and avoid soap. Instead, use a cleanser that is safer for your body.

230.   You should always use sunscreen. This is even more important when you have eczema. Use a sunscreen with an SPF of at least 30 so you don't get a sunburn. Having a sunburn can make your skin even itchier than usual. You could use sunscreens specifically formulated for the face on the entire body. These are generally more gentle to use.

231.   Lotions and creams do not usually work as well as ointments. Ointments have a bit more oil in them, which generally helps them moisturize more effectively. They are a little harder to apply than creams, however, but they are much better at adding a protective layer to the skin and easing your symptoms.

232.   If the air in your room is too dry, it may cause your eczema to act up. Therefore, a humidifier is often an important addition to an eczema sufferer's home. Consider which rooms you spend the most time in and place the humidifier there. You should notice a difference in your skin.

233.   Avoid stress. Stress can increase the intensity of eczema flare-ups. While it is true that eczema itself can stress you out, try not to let it. Practice relaxation methods like yoga, medication, and deep breathing exercises. Staying calm is your best defense when it comes to successfully battling your eczema.

234.   Choose ointments when you are looking for a moisturizer. These are often more successful at soothing eczema due to their ability to better seal in the moisture. Creams and lotions do not hold in moisture like ointments do. That is why ointments are your best choice when you are dealing with damage from eczema.

235.   One effective skin care regimen which will reduce flare-ups and improve response to medication and treatment is proper application of moisturizers. Moisturizers trap moisture in the skin, so applying moisturizers no later than 3 minutes after bathing is highly effective. Of course, it is still

important to continue to apply a moisturizer to very dry patches of skin throughout the day.

236.   Be gentle when dealing with your eczema. This means only gently drying your skin and gently applying your moisturizer. Your skin is compromised and very sensitive. To keep your soft and supple, you need to treat it with a gentle touch. Avoid friction, scratching, and exfoliating. You should also avoid using harsh bathing items like loofah sponges and shower puffs.

237.   Don't partake in hot showers. They always feel great, but can irritate very sensitive skin. If you suffer from eczema, limit how many hot showers you decide to partake in. Instead you should take a shower with water that is the same temperature as the room. Gently clean skin with a gentle cleanser and moisturize after.

238.   Make sure the air is not too dry in your home, especially in the rooms you spend most of your time in. Dry air can cause break outs of eczema. If it is the heating season or you have particularly dry air in your home, you can fix that by putting a humidifier in those rooms.

239.   Instead of scratching, try using ice to cool itchy areas. You can get an inexpensive gel compress and

keep it in the freezer. Take it out and hold it over itchy areas whenever you need to. Keep a dry washcloth in your purse or pocket at all times. If you become very itchy away from home, soak the cloth in cold water. Hold it over the itchy area.

240.   During the summer months, beware of which sunscreens you use if you have eczema. Every eczema sufferer has certain triggers, but sunscreen lotions are a common one. If you try multiple sunscreens and every one of them seem to cause a flare-up, you may want to chat with your doctor about a prescription alternative.

241.   If you have eczema occasionally, an outbreak may be related to other things that cause allergies. Avoid using strong household chemicals as much as possible, as well as perfumed laundry products. Take care to notice if any type of pattern develops that may associate an outbreak with any of these products.

242.   You may already know to change your sheets frequently but have you considered your curtains? Your curtains can attract a great amount of dust over time and that dust is released in the air whenever you open and close them. So you should wash them frequently or invest in some that are easier for you to wash.

243.   If you are taking a bath, using bath oil or
       scented beads that contain oils are a great way to
       help soothe dry and scratchy skin. Your skin will
       absorb the moisture from the bath and the oils will
       help your skin to retain that moisture and protect
       your skin from drying out.

244.   You definitely want to be sure that you're
       moisturizing your skin often, at least three times
       daily. This is necessary not only for the skin that is
       dry and itchy but also for other skin areas for a
       prevention method. Be sure that you select a
       moisturizer that does not contain added chemicals,
       so go all-natural, and get an unscented product as
       well.

245.   Be sure to keep your skin clean. It is alright to
       bathe every day or even more often. It helps reduce
       itching by removing allergens and adding moisture.
       Additionally, soaking in a warm bath is a great way
       to reduce stress. So is taking a relaxing shower.
       Follow up with a great, natural moisturizer to
       soothe your skin.

246.   Make your moisturizer your best friend. Every
       time you wash your hands or take a bath, apply the
       moisturizer. Do not get fancy. Anything that has a
       scent attached to it could exacerbate your condition.

Also, look for a very thick product to get the best results for your skin.

247.   Your body temperature could have an impact on your eczema. Being too hot could cause you to sweat, which makes the skin irritated and itchy. In the winter time, the humidity inside is quite low, which could cause the skin to dry out and become itchy. Keep these things in mind as to what could make your eczema flare up.

248.   Be careful when you put on sunscreen. You never know what may cause you to have an outbreak of eczema. The higher the SPF, the more likely it is that the sunscreen may cause you to have an issue. Try and find something with an SPF of around 35. That should protect your skin from the sun and keep it in good shape overall.

249.   There are several medications you can try to help relieve the itching of eczema. Topical treatments including calamine lotion, which helps soothe the itching. Another topical option is an over-the-counter cream that contains one percent hydrocortisone. For severe itching, consider an oral over-the-counter antihistamine, such as Benadryl. Follow the instructions on the package, and remember that antihistamines may cause drowsiness.

250.   Try to be aware of anything that triggers your eczema. Flare ups of eczema can be particularly unpleasant. It is important to know what makes your eczema worse. Do scented soaps or lotions aggravate your skin? Make note of anything that causes your eczema to flare up, and make a point to avoid it.

251.   Some types of clothing can be a real irritant to your eczema. Fabrics, such as synthetics, can make eczema flares come alive. People with eczema should wear cotton. Also, be sure to wash new articles of clothing prior to wearing them. Use a liquid detergent that's mild, unscented, and without a fabric softener when you clean your clothes.

252.   Try to limit how much you sweat to prevent eczema flares. Prolonged sweating can exacerbate your eczema symptoms. If you are the active type, cool your body down soon after you are done with your physical exertion. If possible, shower immediately after exercising.

253.   Remember to moisturize your skin. Moisturizing your skin regularly is one of the best ways you can combat eczema. Look for thick, unscented moisturizers that will not aggravate your skin. Too many chemicals or additives in a moisturizer can be

counterproductive. Apply it on a daily basis, especially after taking a shower or bath.

254.   Keep your hands protected. These eczema-prone areas are exposed to water and irritating substances like cleaning products. Too much moisture or sweat can trigger symptoms. When you need to submerge them in water, try using rubber gloves. Wearing cotton gloves can also keep hands protected when doing work around the house. Try wearing cotton or leather gloves when doing outside work.

255.   A humidifier can be quite helpful. They will help emit steam in the air. This moisturizes the air around you. This can keep skin healthy through all seasons. Also, cleanliness of the humidifier will keep you healthy.

256.   Make sure the air is not too dry in your home, especially in the rooms you spend most of your time in. Dry air can cause break outs of eczema. If it is the heating season or you have particularly dry air in your home, you can fix that by putting a humidifier in those rooms.

257.   The clothing you wear can affect whether or not you have eczema flare-ups. Those with eczema should wear clothing made of cotton or cotton

blend. On the other hand, clothing made of synthetic fibers and wools ought to be avoided, as they can irritate your skin. Also, wash any clothing your purchase before wearing it.

258.   Try to wear gloves throughout the day to prevent dryness. It is essential that your hands be protected. When you are washing dishes by hand, put on rubber gloves to prevent irritation. When you do chores, wear cotton gloves, and wear leather gloves in the cold. Wool fabric close to the skin should be avoided. It may cause issues with your eczema.

259.   Taking care of your mattress is important too. Your mattress will accumulate dead skin cells, dust, dust mites and other irritating particles. This is why you need to vacuum your mattress on a regular basis to keep those irritants to a minimum. After all, one third of your life is spent in your bed so it need to be a safe zone.

260.   Eczema sufferers can benefit from cutting their nails regularly. This will reduce the effects if you were to itch. However, long, dirty nails being used to scratch your skin may cause infections. Prevent that from occurring by keeping your nails short and clean.

261.   Be cautious with your use of perfumes and fragrances. Fragrances can be one of the biggest triggers for allergy or eczema outbreaks. Many fragrances contain the same chemical so you may have to try a more natural fragrance such as essential oils if you want to have a nice smell without the chemicals.

262.   Make sure you make good use of humidifiers. Dry air makes eczema worse. Their skin can get flaky and begin to itch. Using a humidifier keeps the air moist, which in turn helps the skin.

263.   One key factor in controlling eczema is to daily practice good skin care. When washing your skin, it's best to use a soap substitute or a mild soap. These cleansing agents are less likely to dry out your skin. Immediately after bathing, always apply a good moisturizer. Moisturizers help conserve your skin's natural moisture.

264.   Common treatments for eczema include topical creams and ointments that contain cortisone. You could try hydrocortisone that can be purchased at your local drug store. If this doesn't soothe your eczema, you should talk with your doctor about possibly getting a stronger prescription from him. These will work like other steroid creams, but will be able to be used for a longer time.

265.   Your body temperature could have an impact on
your eczema. Being too hot could cause you to
sweat, which makes the skin irritated and itchy. In
the winter time, the humidity inside is quite low,
which could cause the skin to dry out and become
itchy. Keep these things in mind as to what could
make your eczema flare up.

266.   Moisturize your skin often. Moisturizers are of
great help when it comes to controlling eczema.
After you bathe, moisturize immediately. You
should only use moisturizer that's free from
fragrance or chemicals. These things can irritate the
skin. Creams or ointments work better.

267.   Learn what triggers your eczema. Some people
get flare up from dust mites, cosmetics, and certain
foods. Even things like grass, soaps, and perfumes
can cause flare-ups. Some items can trigger
symptoms in almost all eczema sufferers like
fragrances and cleaning products. When you learn
what items make your symptoms worse, try to stay
away from them.

268.   Use an antibiotic ointment on severely cracked
skin. This can prevent infections from forming. It
also serves as a moisturizer. Do this sparingly
though; prolonged use of antibiotic ointments can

render them ineffective. If you do have an infection, you should consult your doctor, who may give you an oral antibiotic.

269.   Make your eczema less itchy by taking a bath that's warm. Make sure the water isn't too hot. Consider using a bit of colloidal oatmeal or baking soda for a soothing bath. It has also been said that adding 1/2 cup or so of bleach to a 40-gallon bath will remove any bacteria from the skin.

270.   Although eczema presently can't be cured, there are various strategies that be used to manage it. If you have eczema on your hands, always cover them with plastic or vinyl gloves when doing water-related chores, such as washing dishes. If you hands tend to sweat while wearing these gloves, wear cotton gloves under them to soak up the sweat.

271.   Be aware of what you're wearing. Garments close to the skin can actually produce eczema flares. Look to anything cotton or blended with cotton. Other fabrics can irritate your skin. Similarly, you need to pay attention to how you wash your clothes. Toss out any chemically laden laundry products.

272.   Know what your eczema is triggered by. For some people, dust mites cause flare-ups. Other people find that scented soaps are problematic.

Make sure that you identify your trigger points that might lead to an outbreak. You may have to change things up, but you won't have to battle with eczema.

273.   Take a bath at least once a day. Showers are great for getting clean, but sitting in the tub is the best way to soothe and moisturize your skin. You do not need to limit yourself to one bath a day. If you find that it helps, take as many baths as you need to.

274.   If you have to use rubber or latex gloves, put on a pair of thin cotton gloves before you put the rubber or latex gloves on. This will help avoid a reaction to the rubber or latex and will help keep your hands protected from the sweat that these gloves can cause.

275.   Have your doctor run some tests to identify any allergies you may have. It is possible your eczema is an allergic reaction to products like gluten, peanuts, soy or dairy. These are common allergens, and it's a good idea to avoid them. Add soothing substances like vitamin A and vitamin D, fish oils, coconut oil and fish oils to your diet.

276.   When you buy new sheets, always wash them first. They may seem clean and fresh but they are likely stiff with starch or other chemicals that can be

irritating to your skin. So give them a wash with a gentle detergent and use an unscented softener to reduce the risk of irritation to your skin.

277.   When taking a bath, don't use excessively hot water. It will dry out your skin which will aggravate your eczema. Use warm water, a gentle soap and a soft rag to clean any patches of eczema that you have. If you really want to use a loofah or a scrubbie then only use it on unaffected areas and rinse, clean and dry the loofah or scrubbie afterwards.

278.   Rinse your laundry a second time. Laundry detergents can be terrible skin irritants. Even if you are already buying and using an unscented laundry detergent intended for sensitive skin, it may still cause your eczema to flare up. Try rinsing your laundry twice, getting as much detergent off your clothes as possible, just to be safe.

279.   If you need a soothing solution for eczema symptoms, look for a moisturizer in ointment or cream form. These are more effective than lotions. Even petroleum jelly is a good way to soothe and soften your skin. No matter the choice, be sure that it's free of fragrances and alcohol. You should apply moisturizer twice a day for best results.

280.   When buying a detergent, look for something that is not scented. If you are having trouble finding one that works for you, look for products labeled "free and clear" and see if they work. In addition, it may be best not to use a fabric softener at all. This product can cause an issue for people with eczema, so it is usually not worth the risk.

281.   The cold weather can damage your skin, particularly the skin on your hands. When you are outside in the winter, make sure you put on a pair of gloves. In particular, either cotton gloves or leather gloves will work the best. Stay away from wool gloves, as they may hurt more than they will help you.

282.   Be careful when you put on sunscreen. You never know what may cause you to have an outbreak of eczema. The higher the SPF, the more likely it is that the sunscreen may cause you to have an issue. Try and find something with an SPF of around 35. That should protect your skin from the sun and keep it in good shape overall.

283.   Know what your triggers are so you can avoid them. Your triggers may laundry detergent, soaps, and dust. You should probably steer clear of any products that contain fragrances, chemicals or other unnatural additives. Choose pure and unscented

products instead. This will help to reduce the discomfort of daily eczema flare-ups.

284.   Those who have eczema should not use a washcloth or body sponge when they are taking a bath or a shower. If you wash your body with such rough-surfaced items, the friction will irritate your skin. Skin irritation can lead to a flare-up of your eczema. To clean your body, simply use your hands to lather up.

285.   Always moisturize your skin to prevent eczema flare-ups. Use this to really get control of those flare-ups. To keep your skin soft and supple, moisturize your skin frequently following your bath or shower. Use plain, unscented moisturizers rather than products that have chemicals and other additives.

286.   There are several things you can do to keep yourself from scratching your eczema. The best thing to do is keep it covered. Loose clothing may work, or try bandages or dressings on the afflicted area. Keep your fingernails trimmed short, and consider wearing gloves when you go to bed to avoid scratching while you are sleeping.

287.   Keep your stress levels down if you have eczema. The chances of having it flare up increase

when you are stressed out. Stress can also make eczema itchier and more uncomfortable. That can create a never-ending cycle of anger and frustration from dealing with both your stress and your skin. Try relaxing by doing activities like yoga, deep breathing, and meditation.

288.   What triggers are causing your eczema to flare up? You may have to look at the colognes, soap, even your laundry soap, all the way to the material you wear to determine what causes problems. Stress and excessive perspiration can also be to blame. Once you know what your triggers are, you can make a plan to stay away from them.

289.   If you have any of the many types of eczema, you should keep your fingernails cut short. Although individuals try to refrain from scratching the patches of dry, itchy skin, sometimes scratching is done as a reflex without conscious though. With shortened nails, it's less likely that the dry, delicate skin will be punctured when you scratch it.

290.   Moisturize your skin immediately after taking a bath. Applying lotion to your skin soon after your bath helps to lock in the moisture and prevents your skin from drying too much. For the best results, use a intensive moisturizer that does not

have added perfumes or dyes, which can dry your skin more.

291.   Do you have a child that has eczema? Even though you have tried to keep you child from scratching areas of skin that are itching, it still happens. To minimize the amount of damage done when they succumb to the itch/scratch cycle, keep your child's fingernails clipped short. To help prevent damaging scratching during sleep, cover their hands with soft, cotton gloves.

292.   Most patients with eczema already know how important it is to moisturize their skin. But, what many do not know is the proper way to moisturize it. For starters, use a product that is unscented and contains no chemicals, as this can bother your skin. Also, be sure to moisturize frequently, especially after you shower.

293.   Use a wet cloth to dust. This helps the dust adhere to the dusting cloth. Dry dusting does not collect the dust and makes the air more polluted which will affect your eczema.

294.   Always wash your bedding, blankets and pillows on a regular basis. Don't wait until they seem dirty. Do it at least once a week to keep you bed as free from allergens and irritants as possible. Use a gentle

detergent and softener that doesn't contain harsh chemicals or fragrances which can cause irritation to sensitive people.